VASCULAR SURGERY NUTRITION PLAN

Complete Guide Unlocking The Secrets Of
Nutrition To Rapid Healing After Surgery
Success, Nourishing Meal Plans, Recipes, Tips
For Optimal Health Wellness)

DR. ALLAN FREDA

Contents

CHAPTER 1 5

INTRODUCTION TO VASCULAR SURGERY AND
NUTRITION 7

CHAPTER 2 12

THE BASICS OF VASCULAR-FRIENDLY INGREDIENTS 12

CHAPTER 3 18

PLANNING MEALS FOR HEART HEALTH......................18

CHAPTER 4 26

BREAKFASTS TO GET YOU GOING 26

CHAPTER 5 35

HELPFUL LUNCHES TO KEEP YOU ENERGISED..................35

CHAPTER 6 44

HEART-HEALTHY DINNERS THAT WILL FILL YOU UP 44

CHAPTER 7 53

SNACKS AND APPETIZERS THAT HELP THE BLOOD
VESSELS..53

CHAPTER 8 59

DESSERTS WITH A CARDIOVASCULAR TWIST 59

CHAPTER 9 65

DRINKS TO STAY HYDRATED AND PROTECT YOUR HEART
....65

CHAPTER 10 72

LIFESTYLE TIPS FOR MAINTAINING VASCULAR WELLNESS
....72

CONCLUSION 77

1. Understanding Vascular Health: The first part of the book talks about how diet affects vascular health and how it affects the healing process after surgery. Readers will learn more about how certain nutrients can help the body heal and lower the risk of problems.

2. Nutrition Guidelines: A full list of the vitamins, minerals, and nutrients that are important for circulatory health will be given. This part will help readers understand exactly which nutrients they need to focus on in their food to speed up the healing process.

3. Healing Recipes: The book has a group of healing recipes that are specially made to meet the nutritional needs of people who have recently had vascular surgery. People who read these recipes will find it easier to stick to their post-surgery diet plan because the food is both healthy and tasty.

4. Meal Plans: Useful meal plans are included to help readers plan their daily meals so that they meet their nutritional needs. These plans think about things like calorie intake, the distribution of macronutrients, and portion sizes to make sure that healing and general health are at their best.

5. Expert Tips: There will be tips from doctors and nurses who specialize in vascular surgery and nutrition throughout the book. These tips cover a lot of ground, such as changes to your food, your lifestyle, and ways to keep your vascular health in good shape over time.

By following the advice in "Optimal Healing: A Vascular Surgery Nutrition Plan," people who have had surgery can take charge of their healing.

This book is a great resource for anyone who wants to learn more about how to heal and stay healthy through nutrition, whether they have just been identified or are getting ready for surgery.

Disclaimer

The information in this book is for informational purposes only and should not replace professional medical advice, diagnosis, or treatment. Always consult your physician or a qualified health provider regarding any medical concerns. Do not disregard professional medical advice or delay seeking it based on information in this book.

The author does not endorse or have affiliations with any mentioned entities. References are for informational purposes only.

Consult your healthcare provider before making dietary or lifestyle changes, especially during recovery from surgery, as individual needs vary.

Results may vary, and the information provided is not guaranteed to produce specific outcomes.

By reading this book, you acknowledge and agree to consult your healthcare provider before implementing any information herein.

For further guidance, consult your healthcare provider or reputable medical websites for reliable information on surgery recovery diets.

CHAPTER 1
INTRODUCTION TO VASCULAR SURGERY AND NUTRITION

Nutrition is very important for staying healthy and happy in general, but it's especially important for people who are going to have vascular surgery.

Both people who are going to have vascular treatment and people who are patients need to have a full understanding of the link between nutrition and vascular health. As we go through this guide, we will talk about how nutrition affects vascular health, what arterial surgery is, and how nutrition affects vascular health.

How to Understand How Nutrition Affects Vascular Health

The vascular system is made up of the arteries, veins, and lymphatic vessels that carry blood and other fluids throughout the body.

A good diet is important for keeping this system healthy. Nutrients from a varied diet are very important for supporting vascular function.

They help keep blood pressure in check, keep blood vessels healthy, and lower inflammation.

In addition, getting enough nutrients is important for helping the body heal itself, which is especially important after arterial surgery.

Not only is nutrition important for vascular health right after surgery, but it is also essential for long-term arterial health.

Poor food choices, like eating too much-saturated fat, salt, and refined sugars, can make vascular diseases like atherosclerosis, peripheral artery disease (PAD), and venous insufficiency worse and make them more likely to happen. On the other hand, eating lots of fruits, vegetables, whole grains, lean proteins, and healthy fats can lower the chance of vascular diseases and improve overall vascular health.

Vascular surgery includes several different procedures used to fix problems with blood vessels, like blockages, aneurysms, and varicose veins. Surgical intervention is often needed to fix these problems, but nutrition is very important for improving the results of surgery and speeding up the healing process.

Patients may gain from nutritional counseling before surgery to make sure they are well-fed and ready for the procedure. This could mean making changes to your diet, making sure you get enough nutrients, and fixing any deficiencies to improve your general health and help your body heal.

During the time before surgery, diet is very important for helping wounds heal, lowering the risk of complications, and speeding up recovery. Getting enough protein, vitamins, minerals, and other important nutrients is important for keeping your energy up, healing tissues, and keeping your immune system working well. Healthcare professionals who take care of people who are going to have vascular surgery should check their nutritional state, keep an eye on what they eat, and make personalised nutrition suggestions to help the surgery go as smoothly as possible.

What you eat affects the health of your arteries

Nutrition has a big effect on the health of your blood vessels because it changes many bodily processes that help vascular illnesses start and get worse. For instance, eating a lot of saturated fats and cholesterol can cause plaque to build up in the arteries, which makes the blood vessels shrink and slows down blood flow.

On the other hand, eating lots of fiber, omega-3 fatty acids, and vitamins has been shown to improve vascular health by lowering inflammation, making lipid profiles better, and improving endothelial function.

In addition to helping keep vascular diseases at bay, nutrition is also very important for controlling vascular conditions and getting the most out of treatment. As part of a full treatment plan, nutritional measures may be given to people who are having vascular surgery to help the surgery go more smoothly, lower the risk of complications, and support their long-term vascular health. To meet specific nutritional needs and improve general health, this could include making changes to the diet, taking supplements, or living a different way of life.

 diet is an important part of vascular health and is a key factor in achieving the best results from vascular surgery. If healthcare workers know how important nutrition is for vascular health, they can take steps to improve patients' nutritional status before, during, and after surgery. This will improve patient outcomes and long-term vascular health.

CHAPTER 2
THE BASICS OF VASCULAR-FRIENDLY INGREDIENTS

Having vascular surgery is often a major turning point in a person's health journey, requiring not only precise medical care but also a complete approach to recovery and long-term health.

A carefully planned nutrition plan designed to support vascular health and speed up healing is a key part of this method. Understanding the basics of heart-healthy foods, like important nutrients, antioxidants, anti-inflammatory foods, heart-healthy fats and proteins, and the role of carbs and fiber in heart health, is the first step in making such a plan work.

Important Nutrients for Healthy Vascular Systems

Nutrition is very important for vascular health because it gives the body the nutrients it needs to repair tissues, keep the immune system working well, and stay healthy generally. Vitamins and minerals, like vitamin C, vitamin E, selenium, and zinc, are very important among these nutrients. Folks know that vitamin C can protect cells from damage. It helps make collagen and makes the walls of blood vessels stronger, which improves the health and resilience of blood vessels.

Another powerful antioxidant, vitamin E helps fight oxidative stress and inflammation, which are major causes of vascular dysfunction and the formation of atherosclerosis.

Selenium and zinc are good for vascular health because they help the immune system work and speed up tissue repair, both of which are important after arterial surgery.

Getting enough of these micronutrients through food or vitamins is important for a quick recovery from surgery and long-term vascular health.

Adding foods that are high in antioxidants and low in inflammation

It looks like antioxidants and anti-inflammatory chemicals could help protect vascular health from the bad effects of oxidative stress and inflammation. Eating a range of antioxidant-rich fruits and vegetables, like cruciferous vegetables, leafy greens, berries, and citrus fruits, can help the body fight oxidative damage and make blood vessels stronger.

In the same way, eating foods that reduce inflammation, such as nuts, seeds, fatty fish, and olive oil, can help control the inflammatory reactions that are linked to vascular pathology.

Eating a variety of colourful plant-based foods not only improves the nutritional value of the diet but also gives powerful anti-inflammatory and antioxidant effects that are important for a speedy recovery after surgery and long-term vascular health.

Sources of fat and protein are very important for vascular health because they affect lipid levels, inflammation, and endothelial function.

Heart-healthy fats, like those in olive oil, nuts, seeds, avocados, and avocados, can help keep cholesterol levels in check and protect against atherosclerosis, a common problem with the arteries.

In the same way, eating lean forms of protein like chicken, fish, beans, and tofu can help repair tissues and muscles after vascular surgery.

Choosing these heart-healthy fats and lean proteins over saturated and trans fats improves vascular health and lowers the risk of problems after surgery.

This creates an environment that is good for healing and long-term cardiovascular health.

As the body's main source of energy, carbs are important for vascular health, but not all carbohydrates are the same.

Choosing complex carbohydrates like whole grains, legumes, fruits, and veggies gives you long-lasting energy and important nutrients while lowering the risk of blood sugar and insulin spikes.

Fiber-rich foods are also good for your gut health and help keep your cholesterol levels in check, which are both important for heart health.

Many foods, like oats, beans, lentils, and fruits like apples and oranges, contain soluble fiber, which can help lower LDL cholesterol and improve heart health. Insoluble fiber, which can be found in whole grains, nuts, and veggies, makes stools bulkier.

This helps keep bowel movements regular and lowers the risk of constipation, which is a common problem after surgery. People can make smart food decisions to help their recovery and long-term heart health if they know the complex roles that carbohydrates and fiber play in vascular health.

the most important parts of a good post-surgery nutrition plan are the vascular-friendly ingredients, which include key nutrients, antioxidants, heart-healthy fats, and proteins, as well as carbs and fiber. By adding these important nutrients to their diet, people who are having vascular surgery can speed up the mending process, lower their risk of complications, and set themselves up for long-term vascular health. Moreover, eating a variety of nutrient-dense foods not only speeds up physical recovery but also improves general health, giving people the tools, they need to start living a healthier, more fulfilling life.

CHAPTER 3
PLANNING MEALS FOR HEART HEALTH

Eating well-balanced meals is very important for keeping your blood vessels healthy, especially after surgery. A meal full of nutrients helps the body heal and keeps problems from happening.

Focus on including foods from different food groups in your meals, like fruits, veggies, whole grains, lean proteins, and healthy fats. These parts give your blood vessels the vitamins, minerals, antioxidants, and fiber they need to work properly.

Vegetables and fruits are great places to get vitamins C and E. These vitamins are antioxidants that keep blood vessels from getting hurt by free radicals. In addition, they have fiber, potassium, and other nutrients that help keep blood pressure in check and improve heart health in general. Including a variety of coloured fruits and veggies in your meals will help you get all the nutrients you need.

Whole grains, like oats, brown rice, quinoa, and whole wheat bread, have complex carbs that are broken down slowly. This keeps blood sugar levels more stable. Also, they have fiber, which helps your body digest food and lowers cholesterol, which lowers the risk of plaque buildup in your vessels.

After surgery, it's important to eat lean proteins like chicken, fish, tofu, beans, and other vegetables to keep muscles and tissues healthy. Also, they have less fatty fat than red meat, which can cause heart disease if eaten in large amounts.

For healthy blood vessels, you need to eat healthy fats like those found in eggs, nuts, seeds, and olive oil. Fish high in omega-3 fatty acids, like salmon and trout, can help reduce inflammation and keep blood vessels flexible. This lowers the risk of blood clots and artery stiffness.

People can support their vascular health and speed up recovery after surgery by including a range of these nutrient-rich foods in their meals.

Controlling your portions is an important part of a vascular surgery diet plan because eating too much can make you gain weight and make heart disease risk factors like high blood pressure and cholesterol worse. Knowing the right serving amounts can help people stay at a healthy weight and improve the health of their blood vessels.

Using visual cues to guess serving sizes is a good way to control your portions. For instance, a helping of lean protein, like fish or chicken, is about the size of a deck of cards. A serving of carbs, like rice or pasta, is about the size of a tennis ball. Adding different kinds of veggies to your meals can help you feel full without adding extra calories.

Using smaller plates and bowls is another way to do it. This can trick the mind into thinking that smaller amounts are enough.

Also, dividing foods into the right amounts before eating can help you avoid eating too much.

Mindful eating can also help you control how much you eat. People who pay attention to their hunger and fullness signals can stop eating when they're full instead of eating out of habit or boredom.

Being aware of serving sizes and paying attention to their bodies' hunger signals can help people stay at a healthy weight and improve the health of their blood vessels.

Tips for Preparing Meals When You're Busy:

People with busy lives who want to stick to a healthy diet after vascular surgery can benefit from planning their meals ahead of time. People can make sure they always have healthy foods on hand by planning and making their meals ahead of time.

This will make them less likely to eat fast food that is high in unhealthy fats, salt, and added sugars.

One way to plan meals ahead of time is to set aside time every week to make a buying list, plan meals, and get ingredients ready. This can include cutting up veggies, cooking grains and proteins, and putting meals into containers so they are easy to grab and go during the week.

Another good way to prepare meals ahead of time is to cook a lot of food at once. Make a lot of a few basic recipes, like soups, stews, or casseroles, and divide them into individual servings to freeze or refrigerate for later use. This lets you make different kinds of meals without having to cook every day.

Getting useful kitchen tools like a food processor, slow cooker, or Instant Pot can make preparing meals easier and enhance the cooking process. When making healthy meals, these tools can save you time and work.

Finally, adding items that can be used in a lot of different recipes can make meal planning easier. During the week, grilled chicken can be added to soups, wraps, or stir-fries to make them healthier and give you more lean protein.

People who have had vascular surgery can still eat well even when they don't have much time by using meal prep methods that work for them.

Changing traditional recipes to make them better for your heart:

For people who want to improve their cardiovascular health after surgery, it is important to change standard recipes to fit a vascular-friendly diet. By making smart changes and swaps, you can still enjoy your favorite foods while also improving your health and vascular function.

One frequent change is cutting down on the salt that is added to recipes. A lot of salt in the diet can lead to high blood pressure and water retention, which puts more stress on the heart and lungs.

Instead of salt, add herbs, spices, lemon juice, or vinegar to food to make it taste better without hurting your heart.

Another change that can be made to food for vascular health is replacing unhealthy fats with heart-healthy ones. If you want to cook, use olive oil or avocado oil instead of butter and margarine.

For spreads, use mashed avocado or hummus instead of mayonnaise or creamy sauces. These choices give you healthy monounsaturated fats that help keep your blood vessels healthy.

It is also possible to make standard recipes healthier by adding more plant-based ingredients. In recipes like chili, stir-fries, and tacos, use beans, lentils, tofu, or tempeh instead of meat to add fiber and lower the amount of saturated fat.

Adding more veggies to recipes can also make them healthier by adding fiber and nutrients and lowering the number of calories they contain. Spinach, kale, carrots, and bell peppers are good veggies to add to soups, stews, and casseroles to make them filling and healthy.

By carefully choosing what to leave out and add, people can change traditional recipes to improve their vascular health without giving up taste or happiness. After vascular surgery, these changes help the body heal and stay healthy in the long run.

CHAPTER 4
BREAKFASTS TO GET YOU GOING

Breakfast foods that are high in nutrients for heart health

Making sure you get the right nutrition after surgery is important for healing and your general health. This is especially true after vascular surgery, where the body's vascular system needs extra help to recover. As the first meal of the day, breakfast sets the tone for the body's energy and nutrition needs throughout the day. Prioritizing nutrient-rich breakfast choices is very important for people who are recovering from vascular surgery to help them heal and keep their vascular health.

Including foods high in vitamins, minerals, and antioxidants that help the heart work better and fix damaged tissues is an important part of a nutrient-rich breakfast for vascular health.

If you are going to have vascular surgery, you should eat a lot of whole grains, fruits, veggies, lean proteins, and healthy fats. Fibre, which is found in whole grains like oats, barley, and wheat, helps keep blood sugar levels in check and is good for your heart. Vitamins, minerals, and antioxidants like vitamin C, vitamin E, and potassium are found in large amounts in fruits and vegetables.

These nutrients are very important for vascular health because they lower inflammation and support blood vessel function.

For heart health, it's important to think about both the nutrient density and the mix of macronutrients in breakfast foods. Including a mix of carbs, proteins, and fats in your diet can help you stay energetic, repair muscles, and keep your blood sugar levels in check.

For instance, eating whole-grain toast with avocado and eggs gives you a mix of carbs, healthy fats, and protein, which helps you feel full and keep your energy up all morning.

Also, eating foods that help blood flow and vascular health is good for people who have recently had vascular surgery. Fatty fish like salmon or trout, nuts, and seeds are all good sources of omega-3 fatty acids.

These acids help lower inflammation and improve blood flow, which is good for the health of your arteries generally. By adding these foods to breakfast choices, like chia seeds to yogurt or smoked salmon to omelettes, you can improve your nutrition and help your body heal after surgery.

Overall, people who are recovering from vascular surgery should focus on nutrient-dense breakfast choices that include a range of whole foods, well-balanced macronutrients, and ingredients that support vascular health.

By making these breakfast decisions a priority, people can help their bodies heal, improve vascular function, and set the stage for long-term health.

In the busyness of daily life, it can be hard to find time for a healthy breakfast. This is especially true for people who are healing from vascular surgery and may not have much energy or mobility.

But making breakfast a priority is important for giving the body the nutrients and energy it needs to heal and stay healthy generally. For busy mornings, quick and easy breakfast ideas that don't take much time to prepare can be very helpful. This way, people can still eat healthily even while they're recovering.

Overnight oats are a quick and easy way to make breakfast. They can be made the night before and then topped with different things to fit your tastes and nutritional needs. By mixing oats with milk or yogurt and adding veggies, nuts, and seeds, you can make a healthy meal that is full of fiber, protein, and important vitamins and minerals. Overnight oats can be kept in packages that are easy to carry, so they are great for people who need to eat in bed or on the couch while they are recovering.

A smoothie is another quick and easy way to start the day. It only takes minutes to make and is full of nutrients that are good for your heart.

A basic smoothie recipe usually calls for fruits, leafy greens, a drink like water, milk, or juice, and a source of protein like Greek yogurt or protein powder. Adding things like flaxseeds, spinach, kale, berries, and flaxseeds makes it healthier by adding vitamins, enzymes, and fiber. Smoothies are a flexible option for people recovering from vascular surgery because they can be quickly changed to fit different tastes and dietary needs.

Grab-and-go foods like whole grain granola bars, pre-made breakfast sandwiches, or single-serve yogurt cups can be helpful for people who don't have much time in the morning.

Even though these choices may not need much preparation, it's important to pick ones that are low in processed foods and added sugars to make sure they fit with a vascular surgery diet plan that focuses on whole, nutrient-dense foods.

Overall, people who are recovering from vascular surgery can keep up a healthy diet without giving up ease or nutrition by focusing on quick and easy breakfast ideas for busy mornings. Planning and adding easy, healthy foods to your morning routine are ways that people can help their bodies heal and improve their long-term vascular health.

Breakfast smoothies and power bowls are good for your blood vessels.

For people who are recovering from vascular surgery, breakfast smoothies and power bowls are flexible and nutrient-dense choices that make it easy to get all the vitamins, minerals, and antioxidants they need in one meal.

These customizable breakfast options can be changed to fit different dietary needs and taste preferences. They also help keep blood vessels healthy and speed up the repair process.

Smoothies are often had for breakfast because they are cool, easy to stomach, and can be made with different ingredients that are good for your heart. Most smoothies start with a liquid base like water, milk, or yogurt. Then they add fruits, veggies, and extra protein or healthy fats. People who are healing from vascular surgery can make their smoothies healthier by adding things like leafy greens, berries, avocados, and nuts or seeds. These foods provide important nutrients and help the heart work better.

In addition to smoothies, power bowls are a hearty and delicious way to start the day. They contain several nutrient-dense foods all in one bowl.

On the bottom of a normal power bowl are whole grains or leafy greens.

 On top are protein sources like eggs, tofu, or lean meats, as well as different kinds of vegetables, nuts, seeds, and healthy fats. Power bowls can be changed to fit different tastes and dietary needs, which makes them a flexible and useful choice for people healing from vascular surgery.

One great thing about breakfast smoothies and power bowls is that they contain a healthy mix of macronutrients, such as carbohydrates, proteins, and fats. This helps you feel full, keep your blood sugar levels in check, and keep your energy up all morning. People can make sure they are giving their bodies the nutrients they need to heal and recover after surgery by eating a range of nutrient-dense foods, like fruits, vegetables, whole grains, and lean proteins.

Also, it's easy to change up breakfast smoothies and power bowls by adding foods that are good for blood flow and vascular health.

Adding flaxseeds, chia seeds, walnuts, and leafy greens increases the intake of important omega-3 fatty acids, antioxidants, and fiber. These nutrients help lower inflammation, improve blood flow, and support general vascular health.

Overall, adding breakfast smoothies and power bowls to a nutrition plan for vascular surgery is an easy and flexible way to help the body heal and improve vascular health in the long run. With a focus on balance and moderation and a range of nutrient-rich foods, people can make the best breakfast choices to help their bodies recover and stay healthy.

CHAPTER 5
HELPFUL LUNCHES TO KEEP YOU ENERGISED

Healthy lunch ideas to help blood vessels work better

It is very important for your health, especially after vascular surgery, that your lunch is both tasty and full of nutrients that help your blood vessels work well. Including healthy foods in your lunch can help your body heal, improve circulation, and give you energy that lasts all day.

A quinoa salad full of colorful veggies like bell peppers, tomatoes, cucumbers, and leafy greens is a great choice for a lunch that is good for your heart. Since quinoa is a very nutritious grain that is high in fiber, vitamins, and important amino acids, it is a great choice for supporting heart health. You can make the salad even healthier by adding lean protein sources like tofu or grilled chicken.

These foods will also keep you full and pleased.

A hearty vegetable soup made with healthy foods like carrots, celery, onions, and beans is another thought for a healthy lunch. Plus, soups are easy to digest, which makes them a great choice for people who are still feeling sick after surgery. Adding plants and spices like ginger, turmeric, and garlic can help reduce inflammation even more, which is good for your health and the health of your arteries.

A Mediterranean-style wrap with hummus, grilled veggies, and avocado is a tasty and healthy choice for people who want something lighter. Wraps are easy to take with you for lunch on the go, and you can change the ingredients to fit your tastes. If you choose whole grain or gluten-free wraps, your meal will have more fiber, which is important for gut health and reducing inflammation.

Adding omega-3 fatty acids to your lunch is also good for the health of your blood vessels. To get more of these heart-healthy fats, try adding fatty fish like salmon or mackerel to your soups or sandwiches. Additionally, for a vegetarian choice, you can add flaxseeds, chia seeds, walnuts, and other plant-based sources of omega-3s to your meals.

 picking healthy lunch meals that support vascular function is important for speeding up recovery and ensuring long-term health after vascular surgery. Adding nutrient-dense foods to your meals, like quinoa, veggies, lean proteins, and omega-3 fatty acids, can help your circulation, lower inflammation, and give you energy that lasts all day. Try out various recipes and ingredients to discover the ones that work best for you. Also, don't forget to get personalized nutrition advice from a doctor or qualified dietitian.

Lunch ideas that you can take to work or on the go
It can be hard to stick to a healthy diet when you have a lot going on, especially for people who are

healing from vascular surgery. You can still eat healthy, filling meals while you're on the go, though, if you plan and prepare them ahead of time. Lunch ideas that are easy to pack and take to work or other activities can help you stay fed throughout the day and keep your blood vessels healthy.

A bento box full of healthy foods like sliced veggies, whole grain crackers, hummus, and lean protein sources like grilled chicken or hard-boiled eggs is a good way to take your lunch with you. Not only do bento boxes look nice, but they are also very useful because they make packing a healthy meal easy. Your favorite foods can be put in your bento box, and you can mix and match different mixtures to keep things interesting.

You can make a mason jar salad ahead of time and take it with you wherever you go for another easy lunch idea. Put hearty veggies like bell peppers, cherry tomatoes, and cucumbers at the bottom of the jar first. Then add leafy greens like spinach or kale.

Put in some protein, like grilled prawns or chickpeas, and finish it off with a tasty vinaigrette sauce. Just shake the jar to spread the sauce out evenly when you're ready to eat, and you can enjoy a fresh, filling salad on the go.

If you're short on time, a smoothie with healthy foods like berries, fresh greens, Greek yogurt, and almond milk can be a quick and easy way to pack a lunch for the go. Invest in a good blender that is easy to move around, and try mixing fruits and veggies in different ways to make smoothies that are both tasty and good for your heart.

Foods that are high in vitamins, minerals, and antioxidants are important to choose for portable lunch ideas because they help with healing and general health. Stay away from processed foods and sugary snacks, which can make inflammation worse and make it harder for blood vessels to work properly.

Choose whole foods instead, which give you long-lasting energy and help your blood flow, so you feel your best all day.

Making movable lunch ideas a part of your daily life can help you eat well while you're on the go, especially while you're healing from vascular surgery. Whether you like smoothies, bento boxes, or salads in mason jars, many easy choices are good for your heart and your health in the long run. Make sure you carefully pack your meals ahead of time so you can enjoy healthy lunches wherever your day takes you.

Salads, wraps, and sandwiches full of ingredients that are good for your arteries

Salads, wraps, and sandwiches are all flexible meal choices that are easy to change up by adding different heart-healthy foods. You can choose from a variety of tasty foods that are good for your heart and help you recover from surgery. These include a light and refreshing salad, a hearty wrap packed with lean proteins and veggies, or a classic sandwich with a healthy twist.

Adding a variety of colorful veggies to salads, like tomatoes, bell peppers, carrots, and cucumbers, is the best way to make them taste better and protect your health. Adding lean protein sources like beans, grilled chicken, or tofu can help you feel fuller and help your muscles heal and fix. For an extra nutritional boost, you could add heart-healthy fats like avocado slices, nuts, or seeds to your salad.

Wraps are another great option for a heart-healthy meal because they are easy to carry and make it possible to enjoy a variety of healthy foods. Choose wraps made from whole grains or without gluten to get more fiber in your food and help your digestive system. Put healthy foods in your wrap like grilled veggies, hummus, lean deli meats, and fresh herbs to make it taste and feel better.

If you're craving a classic sandwich, try replacing some of the normal ingredients with ones that are better for your heart. Instead of bland white bread, choose whole grain bread or wraps to get more fiber in your meal and feel fuller for longer. Add turkey, chicken, or tuna, which are all lean sources of protein, to your sandwich. For extra nutrition, add spinach, lettuce, tomatoes, and onions.

For healthy blood vessels, adding omega-3 fatty acids to your soups, wraps, or sandwiches is also a good idea. To get more of these heart-healthy fats, you could eat more fatty fish like salmon or mackerel or plant-based foods like flaxseeds, chia seeds, or walnuts. Researchers have found that omega-3s lower inflammation, improve circulation, and support heart health in general. This makes them an important part of a diet that is good for your heart.

salads, wraps, and sandwiches are all flexible meal choices that are easy to change up by adding different heart-healthy foods. No matter, if you like a light and refreshing salad, a filling wrap, or a classic sandwich, many tasty and healthy foods, can help you heal and stay healthy after vascular surgery. Try putting together different combinations of ingredients to see what works best for you. Then, enjoy meals that are healthy, filling, and good for your heart and general health.

CHAPTER 6
HEART-HEALTHY DINNERS THAT WILL FILL YOU UP

Delicious dinner recipes to help your blood vessels stay healthy

When it comes to meal plans for people who are having arterial surgery, dinner is very important. This is the time of day when we relax, give our bodies a break, and get ready for a good night's sleep. For this reason, making tasty dinner recipes that not only please the taste buds but also help keep blood vessels healthy is important for general health.

When recovering from vascular surgery, what you eat is very important for helping you heal and avoiding problems. It is very important to choose foods that are high in nutrients that are good for your heart. Leafy veggies, lean proteins, whole grains, and healthy fats are some of the foods that can help you recover the best after surgery. Not only do these ingredients taste great, but they are also full of antioxidants, vitamins, and minerals that help the body heal and lower inflammation.

It's important to keep balance and moderation in mind when making dinner recipes for vascular health. A range of nutrient-dense foods should be eaten at each meal to make sure the body gets all the nutrients it needs for healing and overall health. It's also important to think about meal sizes since eating too much can put extra stress on the vascular system and slow down the healing process.

If you want to improve your heart health through dinner recipes, there are many tasty choices. Herbs and spices that are good for your heart, like garlic, mustard, and ginger, can make food taste better and be better for you in other ways. These ingredients are known to help reduce stiffness and speed up recovery after surgery because they are anti-inflammatory.

Focusing on lean protein sources like fish, chicken, tofu, and legumes can also give your body the amino acids it needs to fix and grow new tissues. By mixing protein-rich foods with fiber-rich veggies and whole grains, you can make well-balanced meals that are good for your heart and general health.

making tasty dinner recipes that are good for your blood vessels requires careful thought about the ingredients and the health benefits of each one. You can make heart-healthy meals that are also satisfying by using a range of nutrient-dense foods, focusing on balance and moderation, and heart-healthy herbs and spices. These can help with recovery from surgery and long-term vascular health.

Meals that only need one pot or a sheet pan make cleanup easy.

After vascular surgery, people often want to save time without giving up nutrients. One-pot meals and sheet pan dinners come in handy here because they are easy to make and clean up, which makes them perfect for people who are following a vascular surgery diet plan.

One-pot meals are great because they are easy to make and can be used in many different ways. These recipes make cooking easier by putting all the ingredients in one pot or pan. They also require less work and cleanup. This is especially helpful for people who are healing from surgery because they don't have to spend a lot of time making meals, which can be stressful.

Additionally, one-pot meals make it easy to include a wide range of healthy foods in a single dish. Because these meals have lean proteins, whole grains, and a variety of veggies, they provide a complete nutritional profile that helps keep blood vessels healthy and speeds up the healing process. One-pot meals are also popular with people who are following a vascular surgery nutrition plan because the flavors can be easily changed to fit personal tastes.

Also, sheet pan dinners are just as simple and convenient, and they're also very easy to clean up afterward. By putting everything on one sheet pan and baking it in the oven, these recipes cut down on the number of pots and pans that need to be used.

This makes cooking faster and easier to clean up. This is especially helpful for people who are limited in their movement or energy after surgery because it makes it easier for them to make healthy meals.

For vascular health, it's important to plan one-pot meals and sheet pan dinners with a focus on food density and balance.

Adding different colors and shapes to food makes it more appealing to look at and also makes sure it is full of vitamins, minerals, and antioxidants that your body needs. Additionally, picking lean protein sources and whole grains gives the body the nutrients it needs for healing and general health.

one-pot meals and dinners made on a sheet pan are very helpful for people who are following a diet plan for vascular surgery. Because they are quick, easy, and clean up after, these recipes make cooking faster and easier, which is good for recovering from surgery.

Focusing on nutrient density and balance can help you make meals that are both filling and healthy for you in the long run.

Comfort foods that are good for your heart for a good night's sleep

We all love comfort foods because they bring us warmth and peace during hard times, like the time it takes to heal after vascular surgery.

Some traditional comfort foods might not be good for you after vascular surgery, but many heart-healthy options can feed your body and mind.

It's important to put heart-healthy items that support healing at the top of your list when making heart-healthy comfort foods for the evening.

To do this, you should eat lots of healthy foods like fruits, veggies, whole grains, and lean proteins, and as little added sugar, saturated fat, and sodium as possible.

A vegetable and bean chili is an example of a warming food that is good for your heart. This food is full of fiber, protein, and antioxidants from tomatoes, bell peppers, onions, bell peppers, and beans. It's a filling and healthy meal that is good for your heart. Also, choosing lean protein sources like tofu or ground turkey lowers the amount of excess fat while still providing important nutrients.

A hearty vegetable and lentil soup is another choice that will make you feel better. This soup has a lot of vitamins, minerals, and fiber that can help you recover from surgery.

 It has veggies like carrots, celery, and spinach that are high in nutrients and lentils that are high in protein.

Adding herbs and spices like thyme, rosemary, and garlic not only makes the food taste better, but it also has health benefits, like lowering inflammation and making the immune system stronger.

There are also heart-healthy dessert choices for people who want to treat themselves without sacrificing their health. One example is a mixed berry crumble made with oats, almonds, and a little honey. It's sweet and filling, and it's full of heart-healthy fats and vitamins. Adding a dollop of Greek yogurt to it adds protein and probiotics, which are also good for your heart.

making heart-healthy comfort foods for relaxing nights means picking items that are good for your blood vessels and help your body recover from surgery. By including foods that are high in nutrients, like fruits, veggies, whole grains, and lean proteins, you can make meals that are satisfying and healthy without sacrificing comfort.

These recipes, like a bowl of vegetable and bean chili, a hearty lentil soup, or a tasty berry crumble, will make you feel good and help your heart stay healthy in the long run.

CHAPTER 7
SNACKS AND APPETIZERS THAT HELP THE BLOOD VESSELS

You can't say enough about how important it is for people having vascular surgery to have a well-structured diet plan. An all-around diet plan not only helps with recovery, but it's also very important for improving vascular health and boosting general health. While there are many parts to a healthy diet, snacks and appetizers play a big role because they let you eat important nutrients while filling cravings and keeping your energy level steady. This part goes into detail about how to make snacks and appetizers that are good for your heart health, including choices that are high in nutrients, heart-friendly gatherings, and effective ways to control your cravings.

Healthy snack options to keep your blood vessels healthy

Nutrient density is the most important thing to think about when choosing snacks to support artery health. Choosing snacks that are high in fiber, healthy fats, vitamins, and minerals can help your heart health in general.

Berry, orange, and apple foods are good for you because they contain antioxidants and fiber that help lower inflammation and improve blood flow. Besides that, nuts and seeds like flaxseeds, almonds, and walnuts contain heart-healthy fats, protein, and fiber that help lower cholesterol and keep arteries healthy.

Protein- and calcium-rich snacks like Greek yogurt and cottage cheese are important for bone and muscle health. Also, eating whole grains like oatmeal or whole-grain bread can give you long-lasting energy and help keep your heart healthy because they are high in fiber.

People can support their vascular system and speed up the healing process after surgery by picking snacks that are high in nutrients.

Small bites and appetizers for events that are good for the heart

At events or social gatherings, serving appetizers that are good for the heart makes sure that people can stay healthy without giving up taste or pleasure. Giving people appetizers that are high in heart-healthy foods not only improves their health, but also creates an atmosphere that encourages them to eat well.

Veggie plates with guacamole or hummus, for example, offer a wide range of nutrients, such as vitamins, minerals, and antioxidants, as well as healthy fats and fiber. Lean protein choices, like grilled chicken skewers or prawn cocktails, also help you feel full and build muscle without having too much-saturated fat. As an appetizer, whole grain bruschetta or small quinoa salad cups are great ways to get complex carbs and fiber into your diet. This is good for your heart and gives you long-lasting energy. Hosts can prioritize their guests' heart health while still making sure they have a satisfying meal by choosing appetizers that are good for the heart.

Snacking smartly is a key part of controlling your hunger, keeping your blood sugar levels steady, and keeping your energy up all day. People with busy lives and demanding schedules may find it easier to stick to their vascular support diet plan if they develop healthy snacking habits.

One important approach is to watch your portions since eating too many snacks can make you eat more calories than you need to and get in the way of your vascular health goals. People can control how many calories they eat while still satisfying their hunger by choosing pre-portioned snacks or cutting up larger amounts into smaller servings.

Also, eating carbs with protein or healthy fats can make you feel fuller and keep your blood sugar from rising too quickly. For instance, eating apple slices with peanut butter or whole-grain crackers with cheese gives you a healthy mix of macronutrients that makes you feel full and gives you energy that lasts.

Also, drinking water throughout the day can help you control your hunger and avoid becoming dehydrated, which can be bad for your artery health. When people use these smart snacking techniques, they can control their cravings, get more energy, and reach their long-term vascular health goals.

Finally, people who are going to have vascular surgery need to make sure they have a well-rounded eating plan that includes snacks and appetizers that are good for their vascular health. People can speed up their recovery and improve their long-term cardiovascular health by choosing nutrient-dense foods first, bringing heart-healthy foods to meetings, and taking smart snacking into account. Focusing on balance, variety, and amount of control can help people feel good about their post-surgery diet, knowing that they are doing everything they can to protect their vascular health.

CHAPTER 8
DESSERTS WITH A CARDIOVASCULAR TWIST

Recipes for sweet treats that are good for your heart:

Giving in to sweets can feel like a sin, especially for people who are on a nutrition plan for vascular surgery. But you can still enjoy sweets while putting your heart health and general health first. Heart-healthy ingredients in sweet recipes are a delicious way to meet cravings without giving up on your nutrition goals. By using foods that are high in vitamins, fiber, and important nutrients, these desserts not only taste great but also help keep your blood vessels healthy.

Heart-healthy ingredients should be a top priority for people who are having vascular surgery or who are dealing with arterial health problems.

These items can be creatively added to daily diets by using them in dessert recipes. For instance, sweets with dark chocolate, berries, nuts, and whole grains are both tasty and good for you.

Dark chocolate in particular is known for being high in antioxidants and possibly being good for your heart. People can enjoy a treat while also improving their heart health by choosing recipes that use high-quality dark chocolate with few added sugars.

Adding fruits like berries to sweets also gives them natural sweetness and a burst of flavor without the need for a lot of extra sugar. Berries are full of phytochemicals, vitamins, and minerals that are good for your heart and lower inflammation. Berries taste better and are better for you when you eat them with Greek yogurt or add them to whole-grain muffins or oatmeal cookies. Nuts like almonds, walnuts, and peanuts also contain healthy fats, protein, and fiber, all of which help you feel full and improve your heart health.

People who are following a vascular surgery diet plan often focus on cutting back on sugar and fat. Treats with less sugar and fat can help you satisfy your sweet tooth while still following healthy eating guidelines. These treats focus on using whole, nutrient-dense foods with little to no extra sugars or unhealthy fats, which is good for your heart and your health in the long run.

Instead of refined sugars, you could use natural sweeteners like honey, maple syrup, or dates to make sweets that are lower in sugar. These other sugars still add to the total amount of sugar, but they have more nutrients and a lower glycemic index than regular sugars. Fruits like bananas, applesauce, or pureed prunes can also be used to make baked goods sweeter and drier without adding extra sugar or fat.

Along with cutting down on sugar, vascular health needs to cut down on unhealthy fats in sweets. If you choose heart-healthy fats like avocado, olive oil, or nut butter, you can make sweets taste and texture better without hurting your health. Essential fatty acids and vitamins found in these fats help the heart work well and lower the risk of inflammation and oxidative stress. When used in place of butter or shortening in recipes for brownies, cakes, or muffins, these choices can make them much healthier while keeping their delicious taste and texture.

Even if you are on a diet plan for vascular surgery, desserts are an important part of satisfying your sweet tooth and making you feel like you deserve to treat yourself. People can enjoy rich sweets without giving up their health goals as long as they focus on using high-quality ingredients and watching their portions.

When it comes to desserts, these put quality over number, focusing on taste, texture, and presentation to make a truly satisfying meal.

Carefully choosing items that are high in both taste and nutrition is an important part of making rich desserts. For instance, choosing organic, fair-trade chocolate with a lot of cocoa will give you a lot of flavor and powerful antioxidants. Similarly, using high-quality ingredients like pure vanilla extract, fresh fruit, and high-quality nuts makes sweets taste better and gives you important nutrients and phytochemicals.

Also, it's important to watch your portions when eating rich desserts as part of a diet plan for vascular surgery. People can fully enjoy the tastes and textures of sweets without overindulging if they take their time and enjoy small amounts.

This method lets you enjoy food more without breaking any rules about what you can eat or your health goals.

Mindfulness-based practices, like Savoring each bite and eating without distractions, also improve the dining experience and help people have a healthier connection with food.

Finally, desserts with a vascular twist are a tasty and satisfying way to enjoy sweets while also improving your general health and vascular health.

People can enjoy sweet treats without giving up their health goals as long as they use heart-healthy foods, cut down on sugar and fat, and practice mindful indulgence. There are many ways to please your sweet tooth while also taking care of your heart health. These include recipes with dark chocolate and berries, treats with less sugar and fat, or carefully made decadent desserts.

CHAPTER 9

DRINKS TO STAY HYDRATED AND PROTECT YOUR HEART

When it comes to vascular surgery diet plans, drinks are very important for staying hydrated and keeping the heart healthy. You can't say enough about how important it is to stay hydrated, especially after surgery when your body may need more fluids.

Some drinks can also give you nutrients and antioxidants that help your blood vessels work better, which is good for your general heart health. That being said, it's also important to be aware of the drinks you drink, since some can be bad for your artery health.

This comprehensive guide looks into the significance of various beverages in the context of vascular surgery recovery, offering insights into refreshing drink recipes, hydrating options, and tips for limiting potentially harmful drinks.

Refreshing Drink Recipes to Support Vascular Function

One of the key aspects of a vascular surgery nutrition plan is incorporating beverages that support vascular function and help in the healing process. Refreshing drink recipes can offer a delightful way to consume essential nutrients and antioxidants while keeping the body properly hydrated. Incorporating ingredients such as fruits rich in vitamin C, like berries and citrus fruits, can provide antioxidants that help combat inflammation and oxidative stress, which are especially beneficial for vascular health. Additionally, incorporating leafy greens such as spinach or kale into smoothies can offer a rich source of vitamins and minerals, including magnesium and potassium, which are important for maintaining Keeping blood pressure at a healthy level and helping the heart work well generally.

Smoothies are an excellent option for those in the recovery phase of vascular surgery, as they can be easily customized to include ingredients that directly target vascular health.

Adding ingredients like flaxseeds or chia seeds can provide a dose of omega-3 fatty acids, known for their anti-inflammatory qualities and ability to support heart health. Furthermore, incorporating herbs like mint or parsley can not only improve the flavor but also provide additional antioxidants and vitamins.

For those looking for a refreshing beverage without the need for a mixer, infused water can be an excellent choice. Simply adding slices of cucumber, lemon, or berries to a pitcher of water can impart subtle flavors while providing hydration and a boost of important nutrients. Herbal teas, such as hibiscus or green tea, can also be enjoyed either hot or cold and offer added benefits for vascular health. Hibiscus tea, in particular, has been shown to lower blood pressure due to its diuretic qualities and high content of antioxidants called anthocyanins.

Hydrating Beverages and Herbal Teas for Heart Wellness

Hydration is paramount for overall health, especially in the setting of vascular surgery recovery. Optimal hydration not only supports the body's healing processes but also adds to heart wellness by keeping blood volume and circulation. Hydrating beverages such as water, coconut water, and electrolyte-rich sports drinks can help replenish fluids lost during surgery and aid in the healing process.

Water is the best choice for hydration, as it is calorie-free and essential for almost every bodily function. Proper hydration is important for maintaining blood viscosity, which is crucial for cardiovascular health. Coconut water, often dubbed "nature's sports drink," is another excellent choice for hydration due to its high electrolyte content, including potassium and magnesium. These electrolytes play a vital role in regulating blood pressure and supporting muscle function, which is especially important during the recovery phase of vascular surgery.

In addition to traditional beverages, herbal teas can also help with heart health and hydration. Herbal teas such as chamomile, ginger, and rooibos offer a range of health benefits, including anti-inflammatory and antioxidant qualities.

Chamomile tea, for example, has been shown to reduce blood pressure and cholesterol levels, while ginger tea can help improve circulation and reduce inflammation, both of which are good for vascular health. Rooibos tea, derived from the South African red bush plant, is rich in antioxidants such as quercetin and aspalathin, which have been linked to better heart health and blood sugar regulation.

While hydration is essential for vascular health, it's equally important to be aware of the types of beverages consumed, especially those high in sugar and caffeine. Excessive consumption of sugary drinks such as soda, fruit juices, and energy drinks has been linked to an increased chance of obesity, type 2 diabetes, and cardiovascular disease.

These beverages can cause spikes in blood sugar levels and add to inflammation, both of which can negatively impact vascular health.

Similarly, excessive caffeine intake, often found in coffee, tea, and certain soft drinks, can have adverse effects on vascular performance. While moderate consumption of caffeine has been associated with some health benefits, including better alertness and cognitive function, excessive intake can lead to increased heart rate, elevated blood pressure, and irregular heart rhythms, all of which can strain the cardiovascular system.

 choosing the right beverages is paramount for supporting vascular health and promoting optimal recovery post-surgery. Incorporating refreshing drink recipes rich in nutrients and antioxidants, hydrating beverages, and herbal teas can aid in the healing process and contribute to long-term heart health. Additionally, being mindful of limiting sugary and caffeinated drinks can help mitigate possible risks to vascular health, ensuring a comprehensive approach to post-surgery nutrition and general well-being.

CHAPTER 10
LIFESTYLE TIPS FOR MAINTAINING VASCULAR WELLNESS

Maintaining vascular wellness is crucial for general health and longevity, especially for individuals who have received vascular surgery or have been diagnosed with vascular conditions. Lifestyle modifications play a major role in supporting vascular health, alongside medical interventions.

By adopting healthy habits and making conscious choices in daily life, people can promote optimal vascular function and reduce the risk of complications. This comprehensive guide explores various lifestyle tips for keeping vascular wellness, focusing on incorporating exercise and physical activity, stress management techniques, and building healthy habits for long-term vascular support.

Incorporating Exercise and Physical Activity into Daily Life

Regular physical exercise is important for vascular health as it helps improve blood circulation, strengthen the heart, and maintain healthy blood vessels. Incorporating exercise into daily life can significantly benefit people recovering from vascular surgery or managing vascular conditions. Activities such as walking, swimming, cycling, and yoga can be especially beneficial as they promote cardiovascular fitness without putting excessive strain on the vascular system. It's important to consult with a healthcare professional before starting any exercise regimen, especially after surgery, to ensure safety and appropriateness. Gradually increasing the intensity and duration of physical exercise can help people build stamina and endurance while minimizing the risk of injury. Adding strength training to your routine can also help improve muscle tone and circulatory health by increasing blood flow and making the heart work less. Including exercise in your daily routine not only improves your cardiovascular health but also makes your life better in general.

How to Deal with Stress for Healthy Vascular

Long-term worry can hurt the health of your arteries, leading to high blood pressure, stiff arteries, and a higher risk of heart disease. So, using good stress-management methods is important for keeping your vascular health in good shape.

Mindfulness meditation, deep breathing exercises, and progressive muscle relaxation are some of the things that can help lower stress and improve relaxation, which can improve the performance of your arteries. Activities that help you relax and have fun, like spending time in nature, doing sports, or hanging out with friends and family, can also be good for your vascular health. It is important to figure out what stresses you out in daily life and come up with good ways to deal with them.

This could mean setting limits, making a list of things to do, and asking for help from family, friends, or mental health workers when you need it.

By healthily dealing with stress, people can improve their vascular health and lower their chance of complications related to vascular conditions.

Getting into good habits is important for long-term vascular health and well-being in general.

This includes eating a healthy, well-balanced diet, staying at a healthy weight, not smoking, and drinking less alcohol. A diet full of fruits, veggies, whole grains, lean proteins, and healthy fats can give you antioxidants, vitamins, minerals, and other nutrients that are good for your blood vessels.

Heart diseases like cholesterol and high blood pressure can be lowered by staying away from processed foods, too much salt, and saturated fats. Keeping a healthy weight through regular exercise and careful eating can also help stop obesity, which is a major risk factor for vascular conditions.

Quitting smoking and staying away from people who smoke are important ways to protect your circulatory health, since smoking damages arteries and raises the risk of cardiovascular disease.

Limiting your alcohol intake to healthy levels can also help keep your blood vessels healthy since drinking too much can raise your blood pressure and make it hard for your heart to work normally. People can support their long-term vascular health and lower their risk of vascular problems by making these healthy habits a priority and making small changes over time.

keeping your arteries healthy takes a broad approach that looks at many aspects of your lifestyle and behavior.

People can improve their vascular health and lower their chance of complications by making exercise and physical activity a regular part of their lives, learning how to deal with stress well, and forming healthy habits that will last. It's important to talk to medical professionals to get personalized help and advice on making and following a vascular fitness plan that fits your needs and situation. People can improve their vascular health and enjoy better general health for years to come if they devote themselves to a healthy lifestyle.

CONCLUSION

This complete guide has given me a lot of useful information about how to improve my diet after surgery for people who have just been diagnosed with circulatory problems. By going into the complicated link between nutrition and vascular health, this guide has shown how important it is to make smart food choices to help with healing and long-term health.

We've talked about the basics of heart-healthy ingredients in each chapter, focusing on the importance of important nutrients, antioxidants, and heart-healthy fats and proteins. We now know how to make meals that are healthy for our bodies, control our amount sizes, and change traditional recipes to fit our new, heart-healthy eating habits. Every meal, from hearty breakfasts to filling dinners and sweet treats, has been carefully chosen to improve vascular health without sacrificing taste or pleasure.

In addition to meals, this guide has also talked about how important healthy snacks, appetizers, and drinks are for keeping your blood vessels healthy. It also talked about how lifestyle choices like regular exercise, managing stress, and making healthy habits can help keep arterial support going for a long time.

This book is a road map for people who are trying to figure out what to eat after surgery. It has healing recipes, meal plans, and expert advice to help your blood vessels work better and improve your general health.

People can start on the path to better health, vitality, and longevity by using the information and methods in these pages.